ISOMETRIC EXERCISE MASTERY

Unlocking Strength, Health, and Fitness for a Stronger You

Adams .U. Morris

TABLE OF CONTENTS

CHAPTER 1

Introduction to Isometric Exercise

In this opening chapter of our book, "Isometric Strength: A Comprehensive Guide to Building Muscular Power and Endurance," we embark on a journey to explore the intriguing world of isometric exercise. This chapter lays the foundation by introducing readers to the fundamental concepts, origins, and the numerous benefits that this unique form of exercise has to offer.

Defining Isometric Exercise
At its core, isometric exercise involves muscle contractions without a change in the length of the muscle or the joint angle. Imagine pushing against an immovable object, like a wall or a door frame; the muscles work hard, but there is no visible movement. This is the essence of isometric exercise. It's a form of static resistance training that challenges your muscles by pitting them against an opposing force.

A Brief History of Isometric Exercise Isometric exercise isn't a recent fitness trend; it has a rich history that dates back centuries. The term "isometric" itself originates from the Greek words "iso" (equal) and "metric" (length). The Greeks, particularly in the realm of sports, recognized the value of isometric training. Wrestlers, for instance, used isometrics to enhance their strength and leverage. In the mid-20th century, isometric exercises gained prominence in physical rehabilitation settings and as part of military training programs.

Benefits of Isometric Training Understanding why isometric exercise has endured through the ages is crucial to appreciating its value in modern fitness. In this chapter, we delve into the multifaceted benefits of isometric training.

1. Strength and Muscle Development: Isometric exercises target specific muscle groups and can be used to build substantial strength. This is particularly valuable for those who may have limited access to weights or equipment.

2. Joint Stability and Rehabilitation: Isometrics can help stabilize joints and facilitate rehabilitation after injuries. This is because they allow controlled, low-impact muscle contractions, reducing the risk of further damage.

3. Time Efficiency: Isometric workouts are efficient; they don't require a lot of time or space. You can perform them almost anywhere, making them a practical option for busy individuals.

4. Improved Mind-Muscle Connection: Isometrics require a high degree of mental focus and concentration. This not only helps with muscle activation but also enhances mindfulness during workouts.

5.   Versatility: Isometric exercises can be adapted for various fitness levels and goals. They can be a stepping stone for beginners or a powerful tool for advanced athletes.

6. Reduced Risk of Injury: Because isometrics involve no joint movement, they put less strain on the connective tissues. This can be advantageous for individuals with joint issues or those recovering from injuries.

7. Blood Pressure Regulation: Isometric exercises have been shown to help regulate blood pressure, making them beneficial for those with hypertension.

Debunking Myths and Misconceptions In this chapter, we also address some common myths and misconceptions surrounding isometric exercise. One of the most prevalent misconceptions is that isometrics are only useful for increasing strength but not muscle size. We'll explore why this is not entirely accurate and how isometrics can indeed contribute to muscle hypertrophy when applied strategically.

Furthermore, we'll tackle the misconception that isometrics are only suitable for a limited range of individuals, such as bodybuilders. Isometrics are inclusive and adaptable, making them accessible to people of all fitness levels and backgrounds.

In essence, Chapter 1 serves as a gateway into the world of isometric exercise. It aims to pique the reader's interest by highlighting the unique qualities and numerous advantages of isometric training. It dispels common misconceptions and sets the stage for the practical guidance and knowledge to come in the subsequent chapters, where we'll delve into the science, techniques, and applications of isometric exercise.

CHAPTER 2

The Science Behind Isometrics

In Chapter 2 of "Isometric Strength: A Comprehensive Guide to Building Muscular Power and Endurance," we delve deeper into the science that underpins isometric exercise. Understanding the physiological and neurological mechanisms behind isometrics is essential for harnessing their full potential in your fitness journey.

How Isometric Contractions Work At the heart of isometric exercise is the concept of muscle contractions without joint movement. When you perform an isometric exercise, your muscle contracts, generating tension, but it doesn't change in length. For example, if you press your hands together in front of you as hard as you can, you're engaging in an isometric contraction. Your muscles are exerting force, but your hands aren't moving. This static tension causes your muscle fibers to fire, leading to a range of physiological responses.

Muscle Fiber Activation

During an isometric contraction,

muscle fibers are recruited and activated to generate force. This recruitment occurs in a specific order, starting with slow-twitch (Type I) muscle fibers and progressively involving fast-twitch (Type II) muscle fibers as the force requirements increase. This recruitment pattern plays a significant role in the strength and endurance gains associated with isometric exercise.

Neuromuscular Aspects of Isometrics Isometric exercise is closely tied to your nervous system. Your brain sends signals to your muscles to contract, and these signals become more efficient with practice. This improved neuromuscular coordination is one reason why people can develop significant strength gains through isometric training.

Muscle Growth and Isometrics One common misconception about isometrics is that they can't lead to muscle growth. In this chapter, we clarify this misconception. While isometrics may not cause muscle fibers to lengthen as in traditional resistance exercises (like bicep curls), they can still stimulate muscle hypertrophy (growth). This is primarily due to the recruitment of fast-twitch muscle fibers and the time-under-tension aspect of isometric contractions.

Blood Flow and Isometrics

Isometric exercises, especially those involving larger muscle groups, can temporarily restrict blood flow. This restriction, known as occlusion, occurs because the muscle contracts but doesn't release. As a result, metabolites like lactic acid accumulate, creating a unique environment that may contribute to muscle growth and endurance improvements.

Hormonal Responses

Isometrics can trigger hormonal responses in the body. For instance, during intense isometric exercises, your body releases adrenaline, which can enhance your strength temporarily. Additionally, the sustained muscular effort of isometrics can stimulate the release of growth hormone, contributing to muscle repair and growth.

Isometrics and Joint Stability

One of the significant benefits of isometric exercise, especially in rehabilitation and injury prevention, is its impact on joint stability. By strengthening the muscles around a joint without subjecting it to excessive movement, isometrics help enhance joint stability, reducing the risk of injuries.

The Role of Isometrics in a Comprehensive Training Program This chapter also highlights how isometric exercises can complement other forms of training. Isometrics can serve as a valuable component in a well-rounded fitness routine. They can be used to target specific muscle groups, correct muscular imbalances, and enhance overall performance.

In summary, Chapter 2 provides readers with a scientific understanding of how isometric exercise works on a physiological and neurological level. It emphasizes that isometrics are not merely an obscure form of exercise but are rooted in sound scientific principles. This knowledge empowers readers to appreciate the potential of isometric training to enhance muscle strength, endurance, and overall fitness. Armed with this understanding, readers are prepared to dive deeper into the practical aspects of isometric training in the subsequent chapters.

CHAPTER 3

Types of Isometric Exercises

In Chapter 3 of "Isometric Strength: A Comprehensive Guide to Building Muscular Power and Endurance," we explore the various types of isometric exercises, shedding light on the distinctions between static and dynamic isometrics, as well as yielding and overcoming isometrics. Understanding these categories is essential for tailoring your isometric workout to your specific fitness goals.

Static vs. Dynamic Isometrics

Static Isometrics: Static isometric exercises involve holding a specific position or posture, exerting force without any visible movement. Think of holding a plank, where you maintain a fixed position for a set duration. Static isometrics are excellent for improving endurance, as they challenge your muscles to maintain a contraction over time. They are particularly useful for core strength, as well as stabilizing muscles around joints.

Dynamic Isometrics: In contrast, dynamic isometrics incorporate movement. However, the key distinction is that the muscle length remains constant during the movement. For example, wall sits, where you lower yourself into a seated position against a wall and hold it, represent dynamic isometric exercise. These exercises offer the benefits of both strength-building and muscle endurance.

Yielding vs. Overcoming Isometrics

Yielding Isometrics: Yielding isometrics involve pushing or pulling against an immovable object, such as pressing your hands against a wall or resisting a partner's force. The goal is to maintain a steady force against resistance. Yielding isometrics are excellent for building strength and muscle endurance, as they require maximal effort over an extended period.

Overcoming Isometrics: Overcoming isometrics involve trying to move an immovable object. For instance, trying to lift an impossibly heavy weight or push a stationary car. These exercises engage your muscles at their maximum capacity. They are particularly effective for building strength, as they recruit a high number of muscle fibers simultaneously.

Isometric Exercises for Different Muscle Groups

This chapter also delves into the versatility of isometric exercises, highlighting their applicability to various muscle groups in the body.

Core and Abdominals: Planks, side planks, and hollow body holds are fantastic isometric exercises for strengthening the core and abdominal muscles. They improve stability and can help alleviate lower back pain.

Upper Body: Wall push-ups, handstand holds, and the classic "pressing against a doorway" exercise can target the chest, shoulders, and triceps effectively.

Lower Body: Wall sits, leg raises, and glute bridges can engage the lower body muscles, including the quads, hamstrings, calves, and glutes.

Back and Shoulders: Holding a resistance band in a lateral raise or pulling against a resistance band anchored at waist height are great isometric options for the back and shoulders.

Isometric Squats: You can perform an isometric squat by lowering yourself into a squat position and holding it, with your thighs parallel to the ground. This targets the quadriceps and glutes.

By understanding the types of isometric exercises and their muscle group specificity, readers can start customizing their workouts based on their fitness goals. For example, if you want to improve core stability and endurance, you might incorporate static isometric exercises like planks into your routine. If your goal is to build upper body strength, yielding and overcoming isometrics like wall push-ups or doorway presses can be integrated.

Moreover, the chapter emphasizes the importance of proper form and alignment during isometric exercises. Regardless of the type or muscle group targeted, maintaining correct posture ensures that you maximize the effectiveness of the exercise while minimizing the risk of injury.

In conclusion, Chapter 3 provides readers with a comprehensive understanding of the diverse world of isometric exercises. It explores the various types of isometrics and illustrates how they can be applied to different muscle groups. Armed with this knowledge, readers are well-equipped to begin crafting their personalized isometric workout plans, which will be further detailed in subsequent chapters of the book.

CHAPTER 4

Getting Started with Isometric Training

Chapter 4 of "Isometric Strength: A Comprehensive Guide to Building Muscular Power and Endurance" serves as a crucial starting point for readers who are eager to begin their isometric training journey. This chapter focuses on the initial steps, including assessing your fitness level, setting achievable goals, and creating a personalized isometric workout plan.

Assessing Your Fitness Level

Before diving into any fitness program, it's essential to assess your current fitness level. This serves as a baseline, helping you understand where you stand and where you want to go. In this chapter, we guide readers through a series of assessments, both physical and mental, to gauge their fitness readiness:

- Physical Assessments: These include tests to measure strength, flexibility, and endurance. For example, you might assess your core strength with a plank test, your flexibility with a simple toe-touch test, and your endurance with a timed wall sit.

- Goal Clarity: It's essential to have a clear understanding of your goals. Are you looking to build strength, increase endurance, or rehabilitate an injury? Having specific objectives will help tailor your isometric training program.

Setting Goals and Objectives

Once you've assessed your fitness level and have a clear vision of your fitness goals, it's time to set objectives. This chapter provides guidance on how to establish SMART goals:

- **Specific**: Clearly define what you want to achieve with isometric training. For instance, instead of saying "I want to get stronger," specify "I want to increase my bench press by 20 pounds in three months."
- **Measurable**: Goals should be quantifiable so that you can track your progress. Using the previous example, you can measure progress by

tracking the weight you can lift.

- **Achievable**: Goals should be realistic and attainable. Setting goals that are too ambitious can lead to frustration and burnout.

- **Relevant**: Your goals should align with your overall fitness objectives. Isometric training goals should complement your broader fitness plan.

- **Time-Bound**: Set a timeframe for your goals. This creates a sense of urgency and helps with motivation. In the above example, the goal has a three-month timeframe.

Creating a Personalized Isometric Workout Plan One of the key takeaways from this chapter is the importance of personalization. Not all isometric workouts are created equal, and what works for one person may not be suitable for another. In this section, we guide readers through the process of crafting their personalized isometric workout plans:

- **Exercise Selection**: Based on your goals and fitness level, select the isometric exercises that will be most effective for you. If you're a beginner, start with basic exercises like planks, wall push-ups, and wall sits.

- **Frequency and Duration**: Determine how often you'll train and how long each session will last. Consistency is key, but overtraining can lead to burnout or injury. Find a balance that suits your schedule and allows for recovery.

- **Progression**: Plan how you will progressively challenge yourself. Isometric training is most effective when you gradually increase the intensity of your exercises. This could involve longer hold times, increased resistance, or more challenging variations.

- **Rest and Recovery**: Understand the importance of rest and recovery in your plan. Muscles need time to repair and grow. Include rest days in your schedule and consider incorporating other forms of exercise to balance your routine.

- **Tracking and Accountability**: Keeping a

workout journal or using fitness apps can help you track your progress and stay accountable to your goals. Regularly assess whether you're making progress toward your objectives.

This chapter emphasizes that isometric training is not a one-size-fits-all approach. It's about tailoring your workouts to your unique needs and aspirations. Whether you're a beginner looking to improve core strength or an athlete aiming to enhance overall power, a personalized plan is the foundation for a successful isometric training journey.

In conclusion, Chapter 4 lays the groundwork for readers to embark on their isometric training adventure. It guides them through the process of assessing their fitness level, setting realistic goals, and creating a customized isometric workout plan. Armed with this knowledge, readers are well-prepared to move forward and begin their practical exploration of isometric exercise in subsequent chapters of the book.

CHAPTER 5

Proper Form and Technique

Chapter 5 of "Isometric Strength: A Comprehensive Guide to Building Muscular Power and Endurance" focuses on the critical aspect of proper form and technique when performing isometric exercises. Understanding and mastering these principles is essential to ensure the effectiveness of your workouts and minimize the risk of injury.

The Importance of Form and Technique Proper form and technique are the cornerstones of safe and effective isometric training. In this chapter, we delve into why form matters:

1. Injury Prevention: Incorrect form during isometric exercises can lead to muscle imbalances, strain, or even acute injuries. Maintaining proper alignment reduces the risk of these issues.

2. Muscle Activation: Proper form ensures that the intended muscle group is engaged to its fullest. Correct muscle activation leads to better results, as you're targeting the right muscles with the right intensity.

3. Efficiency: Correct technique maximizes the efficiency of your workouts. When you perform an isometric exercise with proper form, you get more benefit from each repetition.

4. Progression: To advance in your training, you need to ensure that you're consistently challenging your muscles. Proper form is vital for understanding when it's time to progress to more challenging exercises.

5. Comfort and Confidence: Correct form helps you feel more comfortable during exercises and boosts your confidence in your ability to perform them safely and effectively.

Key Elements of Proper Form and Technique This chapter explores the fundamental elements that constitute proper form and technique during isometric exercises:

1. Posture and Alignment: Maintaining a neutral spine, keeping your head in line with your body, and aligning your joints correctly are vital components of proper posture and alignment. These principles are crucial for exercises like planks and wall sits.

2. Breathing Techniques: Understanding when and how to breathe during isometric exercises is essential. Proper breathing helps stabilize your core and maintain muscle engagement. We explain techniques such as diaphragmatic breathing and the Valsalva maneuver.

3. Muscle Engagement: Isometric exercises require deliberate muscle engagement. We detail how to "squeeze" or contract the targeted muscle group effectively to generate the required force.

4. Concentration and Mind-Muscle Connection:

Concentrating on the muscle you're working is a fundamental aspect of proper technique. This mind-muscle connection enhances muscle engagement and can lead to better results.

5. Avoiding Common Mistakes:

We address common mistakes that people make during isometric exercises and provide tips on how to correct them. For instance, in planks, the sagging of the hips is a common mistake that can be rectified by engaging the core muscles and maintaining a straight line from head to heels.

Illustrations and Visual Guides: This chapter is complemented with visual aids, such as illustrations and photographs, demonstrating correct form and technique for various isometric exercises. Clear visuals help readers understand and visualize how to perform each exercise correctly.

Progression and Form Checks: We emphasize the importance of continually assessing and refining your form as you progress in your isometric training. What was correct form for you as a beginner might need adjustment as you become more advanced.

By the end of Chapter 5, readers will have a comprehensive understanding of how to perform isometric exercises with precision and safety. They'll grasp the significance of proper form and technique and be equipped with practical knowledge to execute exercises effectively. This foundational knowledge will be invaluable as they progress through their isometric training journey, ensuring they achieve their fitness goals while minimizing the risk of injury.

CHAPTER 6

Equipment and Tools for Isometric Workouts

Chapter 6 of "Isometric Strength: A Comprehensive Guide to Building Muscular Power and Endurance" delves into the equipment and tools that can enhance your isometric training experience. This chapter aims to provide readers with an understanding of the various options available, from bodyweight exercises to specialized isometric devices.

The Simplicity of Bodyweight Exercises The chapter begins by emphasizing the simplicity and accessibility of bodyweight exercises. Bodyweight isometrics require no additional equipment; they rely solely on your body's resistance against gravity. Exercises like planks, wall sits, and handstand holds can be performed anywhere, making them ideal for those who prefer minimalist workouts or who may not have access to specialized equipment.

Incorporating Everyday Objects This section explores creative ways to incorporate everyday objects into your isometric workouts. Common items such as chairs, walls, door frames, and towels can be repurposed as exercise aids. For instance, using a towel to create resistance during isometric shoulder exercises or using a sturdy chair for tricep dips.

Isometric Devices and Tools
Chapter 6 introduces readers to a range of isometric devices and tools that can add variety and intensity to their workouts. These include:

1. Isometric Bands: These elastic bands provide resistance in various directions, allowing you to engage different muscle groups effectively. Isometric bands are versatile and can be used for both upper and lower body exercises.

2. Isometric Bars: Isometric bars are portable and adjustable devices that can be used for exercises like chest presses, leg presses, and more. They provide a stable base for isometric contractions and can be easily stored when not in use.

3. Hand Grippers: Hand grippers are specialized tools designed to improve grip strength. They can be beneficial for athletes in sports like rock climbing or martial arts.

4. Isometric Platforms: These stable platforms are used for exercises like wall sits and are designed to support your body weight while you focus on muscle engagement.

5. Suspension Trainers: Suspension trainers, like TRX systems, can be adapted for isometric exercises by holding static positions while suspended. These versatile tools engage multiple muscle groups and challenge stability.

6. Stability Balls: Stability balls can be incorporated into isometric workouts to introduce instability, which forces your muscles to work harder to maintain balance. They are particularly effective for core exercises.

7. Isometric Machines: For those who have access to a gym or specialized equipment, isometric machines like the isometric leg press or chest press provide controlled and measurable resistance.

Choosing the Right Equipment The chapter offers guidance on how to select the right equipment based on your fitness goals and available space. It emphasizes the importance of aligning your equipment choices with your training objectives and budget.

Safety Considerations Chapter 6 also addresses safety considerations when using isometric devices and tools. It underscores the importance of proper setup, supervision (when necessary), and gradual progression to avoid injury.

Complementary Nature of Equipment and Bodyweight Exercises The chapter emphasizes that equipment is a valuable addition to an isometric training program but should not replace bodyweight exercises entirely. The two can complement each other effectively. For example, using isometric bands to add resistance to bodyweight squats or combining hand grippers with push-ups for a comprehensive upper body workout.

By the end of Chapter 6, readers will have a comprehensive understanding of the equipment and tools available for enhancing their isometric workouts. They'll appreciate the versatility and accessibility of bodyweight exercises, as well as the potential benefits of incorporating various isometric devices and tools into their training routines. Armed with this knowledge, readers can make informed choices about the equipment that aligns with their fitness goals and preferences as they progress through their isometric training journey.

CHAPTER 7

Progressive Overload and Periodization in Isometric Training

Chapter 7 of "Isometric Strength: A Comprehensive Guide to Building Muscular Power and Endurance" is dedicated to two essential principles in effective isometric training: progressive overload and periodization. These principles are crucial for maximizing gains, preventing plateaus, and ensuring a well-structured and sustainable workout routine.

Understanding Progressive Overload Progressive overload is a foundational principle in strength and muscle development, and it's equally crucial in isometric training. This principle involves continually increasing the demand on your muscles over time to stimulate growth and strength gains. In this chapter, we explore how to apply progressive overload to isometric exercises effectively.

1. Increasing Time-Under-Tension (TUT): One way to progressively overload isometric exercises is by extending the duration of the contraction. For example, if you can hold a plank for 30 seconds, aim to increase it to 40 seconds, then 50, and so on. This gradually increases the challenge on your muscles.

2.   Intensity   Variation: Progressive overload also involves making the exercises more challenging. For example, you can increase resistance by using isometric bands or perform more challenging variations of exercises. For instance, moving from wall push-ups to standard push-ups.

3. Incorporating Additional Weight: Some isometric exercises can incorporate additional weight, such as weighted vests or dumbbells. This added resistance increases the challenge and promotes muscle growth.

4. Changing Angles and Positions: By altering the angles or positions in which you perform isometric exercises, you can target muscle groups differently. For example, adjusting your hand placement during a wall push-up can shift the emphasis from chest to triceps.

Understanding Periodization

Periodization is a systematic approach to organizing your training program into different phases or cycles. This helps prevent plateaus, reduce the risk of overtraining, and optimizes performance gains. In this chapter, we explain how periodization can be applied to isometric training.

1. Phases of Periodization: Periodization typically involves three main phases: the **macrocycle** (the entire training program), the **mesocycle** (a specific training phase within the macrocycle), and the **microcycle** (a shorter training cycle, usually a week).

2.   Muscle   Confusion: Periodization involves changing variables such as exercise selection, intensity, volume, and rest periods. This "muscle confusion" prevents your body from adapting too quickly to a single routine, keeping progress steady.

3.   Deloading   Weeks: Periodization often incorporates deloading weeks, during which you reduce training intensity and volume. This allows your body to recover fully and prepares it for more intense phases.

4. Specialization Phases: Periodization can include specialization phases where you focus intensely on specific muscle groups or movements. For example, if you're an athlete, you might have a phase focused on enhancing your core strength for improved performance.

Implementing Periodization in Isometric Training In this chapter, readers learn how to design their periodized isometric training programs:

1. Goal Identification: Identify specific goals for different phases. For instance, one phase might focus on strength, while another emphasizes endurance or muscle hypertrophy.

2. Exercise Selection: Choose isometric exercises that align with your goals for each phase. For strength, focus on more intense and shorter-duration exercises, while for endurance, opt for longer holds.

3. Reps, Sets, and Rest: Determine the number of sets, reps (or hold times), and rest intervals based on your phase-specific goals. For instance, during a strength phase, you might perform fewer reps but with maximal effort and longer rest periods.

4. Tracking and Adjusting: Keep detailed records of your workouts to monitor progress. Adjust your program as needed to ensure continued growth and prevent stagnation.

By the end of Chapter 7, readers will have a solid understanding of how to implement progressive overload and periodization in their isometric training programs. These principles are essential for maintaining motivation, preventing plateaus, and achieving long-term success in isometric training. Armed with this knowledge, readers can approach their workouts with a structured and strategic mindset, optimizing their efforts and results.

CHAPTER 8

Isometrics for Specific Goals

Chapter 8 of "Isometric Strength: A Comprehensive Guide to Building Muscular Power and Endurance" is a pivotal section that dives deep into tailoring isometric training for specific fitness goals. It's in this chapter that readers learn how to customize their isometric workouts to meet their unique objectives, whether it's building strength and power, enhancing muscular endurance, or focusing on rehabilitation and injury prevention.

Building Strength and Power with Isometrics

Building Strength: The chapter starts by elucidating how isometric exercises are a potent tool for building muscle strength. Isometrics can activate a high percentage of your muscle fibers, leading to substantial strength gains. For individuals seeking to increase their raw power, isometrics offer several advantages:

1. **Maximal Contraction:** Isometric exercises allow you to generate maximum force, such as trying to lift an immovable object. This is especially useful for building maximal strength.

2. **Neuromuscular Adaptations:** Isometrics help improve neuromuscular coordination, enhancing the efficiency with which your brain signals your muscles to contract.

3. **Minimal Risk of Injury:** Isometrics impose less stress on the joints compared to dynamic exercises, making

them a safer option for intense strength training.

Building Power: The chapter also delves into how isometric exercises can contribute to power development. Power is the ability to generate force quickly, which is crucial in sports like sprinting, jumping, or explosive weightlifting. Isometric exercises can enhance power in several ways:

1. **Rapid Force Generation:** Isometrics, when performed explosively, help improve the rate at which force is

produced, which is essential for power-based activities.

2. **Stabilization Strength:** Isometrics strengthen stabilizing muscles, enhancing your ability to control and transfer power efficiently during explosive movements.

3. **Sports-Specific Power:** Isometrics can be customized to mimic the demands of specific sports, helping athletes develop power that's directly applicable to their activities.

Enhancing Muscular Endurance

The chapter transitions to discuss how isometric training can be tailored for those who wish to enhance their muscular endurance. Muscular endurance is the ability of a muscle or muscle group to perform repeated contractions over an extended period. Here's how isometrics can be applied to improve endurance:

1. **Time-Under-Tension (TUT) Variations:** Isometrics can be adjusted to increase TUT, gradually enhancing muscular

endurance. For example, you can hold an isometric exercise for longer durations, such as a plank, to build endurance.

2. **Circuit Training:** Isometric exercises can be incorporated into circuit-style workouts, where you move from one exercise to another with minimal rest. This approach improves cardiovascular endurance in addition to muscular endurance.

3. **Specific Muscle Group Targeting:** Tailoring isometric exercises to target

specific muscle groups can be particularly beneficial. For example, isometric wall sits can be used to strengthen the quadriceps, enhancing endurance for activities like cycling or running.

Rehabilitation and Injury Prevention

The chapter also explores the role of isometrics in rehabilitation and injury prevention. Isometric exercises offer a unique advantage in these contexts:

1. **Low-Impact Rehabilitation:** Isometrics allow individuals recovering from injuries to engage their muscles without subjecting their joints to high-impact forces. This can be crucial in early stages of recovery.

2. **Strengthening Weak Muscles:** Isometrics are effective for targeting and strengthening specific muscle groups, which can help correct muscle imbalances and reduce the risk of reinjury.

3. **Improved Joint Stability:** Isometric

exercises enhance joint stability by strengthening the muscles around them, reducing the likelihood of joint-related injuries.

The chapter provides examples and guidance on how to adapt isometric exercises for various rehabilitation scenarios, such as knee injuries, lower back pain, or shoulder issues.

Designing Goal-Specific Isometric Workouts

To conclude the chapter, readers learn how to design isometric workouts tailored to their specific goals:

1. **Exercise Selection:** Choose isometric exercises that align with your objectives. For strength, focus on intense contractions with shorter hold times, while for endurance, opt for longer holds with lower intensity.

2. **Progression:** Apply progressive overload principles relevant to your goal. This might involve increasing the intensity,

duration, or resistance of your isometric exercises.

3. **Periodization:** Implement periodization strategies that match your goal. For example, a strength-focused phase might have shorter rest intervals and higher resistance, while an endurance phase could have longer holds and less resistance.

4. **Rest and Recovery:** Understand the importance of adequate rest and recovery for your chosen goal. Balance your training with rest days and proper

nutrition to support your specific objectives.

By the end of Chapter 8, readers have gained the knowledge and tools needed to adapt their isometric training to their precise fitness goals. Whether they aim to build strength and power, enhance endurance, or focus on rehabilitation and injury prevention, this chapter equips them with a clear roadmap to create effective and goal-specific isometric workout routines.

CONCLUSION

Unleashing the Power of Isometric Strength

In the pages of "Isometric Strength: A Comprehensive Guide to Building Muscular Power and Endurance," we have embarked on a transformative journey into the world of isometric exercise. This book has been your guide to understanding, mastering, and harnessing the remarkable potential of isometrics for a wide range of fitness goals and needs.

Isometric strength is not just a fitness trend; it's a timeless and scientifically-proven approach to building a healthier, stronger, and more resilient body. Throughout this comprehensive guide, we have explored the fundamental principles, techniques, and applications of isometric training, ensuring that you are equipped with the knowledge and tools to take control of your fitness journey.

From the foundational chapters that introduced you to the science and history of isometric exercise to the practical insights on form, equipment, and goal-specific training, this book has empowered you with the wisdom to customize your workouts for your unique aspirations.

Whether your aim is to build muscle strength and power, enhance muscular endurance, or recover from injury, isometric training offers a versatile and effective solution. You've learned to apply progressive overload and periodization strategies, allowing you to break through plateaus and continually advance toward your goals.

Moreover, you've discovered the adaptability of isometric exercises, from the simplicity of bodyweight workouts to the versatility of specialized tools and equipment. You've seen how isometrics can be seamlessly integrated into your fitness routine, whether you're at home, in the gym, or even in the process of rehabilitation.

But beyond the physical gains, isometric strength training has equipped you with mental fortitude. The mindfulness required to maintain proper form, the discipline to push through the intensity, and the patience to see progress—all these qualities cultivated through isometrics extend far beyond the gym.

As you close this book, remember that your fitness journey is a continuous path of growth and self-improvement. Isometric strength training is a lifelong companion that can evolve with you, adapt to your changing goals, and stand by you in your pursuit of optimal health and fitness.

So, take what you've learned here and apply it with dedication and enthusiasm. Whether you're an athlete seeking peak performance, a fitness enthusiast chasing a stronger physique, or someone on a journey to better health, isometric strength can be your steadfast ally.

In your hands now lies not just a book, but a transformative tool to unlock your potential and embrace the enduring power of isometric strength. May your path be strong, your progress steady, and your journey a testament to the remarkable capabilities of the human body and spirit.

www.ingramcontent.com/pod-product-compliance
Lightning Source LLC
Chambersburg PA
CBHW060751260726
48660CB00002B/575